Aromatherapy:

Essential Oils and Healing

By

Debra Helton

ISBN-13: 978-1495915420

Table of Contents

Aromatherapy: Essential Oils and Healing

By Debra Helton

© Copyright 2013 Debra Helton

First Published, 2013

Printed in the United States of America

Introduction

Essential oils are also called essences because they are plant extracts or they are the essences of certain plants but it does not necessarily mean that these oils have an oily feel. Most of the time, these essential oils are used either topically by applying it on the skin or through aromatherapy by inhaling its steam and the aroma that they produce. Essential oils are used for aromatherapy massages as well as medicinal purposes. This is because these oils have healing properties. Whether they are used for massages or for medicinal purposes, their healing properties are activated and can give several benefits to people.

This book Aromatherapy: Essential Oils and Healing will show you health benefits and uses of various essential oils.

Chapter 1. Essential Oils and Their Benefits in Healing

The healing benefits of essential oils range from physical to psychological.

First, essential oils can fight off infectious diseases whether they are caused by bacteria or fungus because these oils have antibacterial and antifungal properties. In fact, they can even fight off diseases caused by viruses and parasites because of their anti-parasitic and anti-virus properties. By applying these essential oils either topically or through aromatherapy, bacteria, viruses and parasites can be killed, thereby healing you from infectious diseases.

Second, essential oils are also good sources of antioxidants. Most of the time, antioxidants are found in plants and since essential oils are extracted from plants, they have antioxidant properties which is a good anti-aging source. Antioxidants have the ability to wash away toxins from the body, thereby paving the way for healthier cells inside the body and a younger looking skin. Third, essential oils are good sources of air purifiers because they usually diffuse a nice aroma. This way, if you are trying to ward off bad odors from your house, essential oils are excellent ways to do so.

Fourth, because of these oils' nice aroma, you are not only capable of purifying the air around you, but you can also bust stress because of their scent. The scent of essential oils is usually strong but nice so aside from the benefits that their aroma can give your home, their aroma can also help you psychologically by getting rid of stress. This is why most people turn to aromatherapy with the use of these essential oils if they want to relax.

Fifth, because of the powerful and healing scent of the aroma produced by these essential oils, it is not only the outer appearance that can benefit from its healing properties but also your respiratory organs. Whatever respiratory diseases you have or any problems with your respiratory organs can be healed. Sixth, these essential oils can also help stimulate blood flow especially when you use them to massage your body, your head or simply inhaling their aroma. This is why they can benefit you a lot by getting rid of aches such as headaches, muscle pains, etc.

Because of the great stimulation of blood flow, they also help the blood distribute oxygen to the body well.

And most of all, essential oils also benefit sleep a lot. They have calming properties that help you fall asleep easily which is why insomnia patients can benefit a lot with these oils.

If you want to reap the benefits of essential oils in your life too, the first step to take is to get to know the different types of essential oils. This way, you'll know what essential oil is best for you or which among the many essential oils are what you need. In fact, the list of essential oils is lengthy. But here are several of the most popular essential oils, their healing properties and how they are best used.

Chapter 2. Different Types of Essential Oils

The Anise Oil. This essential oil does not only have cheering ability but it also heals flatulence, heartburn, gastritis, abdominal pain, stomach ache, and a variety of digestive problems. It also heals respiratory problems like flu, bronchitis and asthma. When exposed in room temperature, this oil solidifies so, it is best used and activated first by simply warming the bottle during your warm water bath. You can either rub the oil to your stomach or inhale its sweet aroma.

The Basil Oil. Basil oil has energizing and refreshing properties as well as it heals digestive and respiratory problems, improves blood circulation, heals infections, treats eye problems, and even gives pain relief. Basil oil works well and is best used with other essential oils like sage, etc.

The Camphor Oil. Camphor oil treats conditions like joint and muscle pain, cough, asthma, colds, rheumatism as well as arthritis. For best effects, use camphor oil as massage oil, for steam inhalation, and blend it with other oils like juniper oil.

The Sage Oil. This oil heals skin diseases, signs of aging like wrinkles, memory loss, etc., wounds, injuries, all types of infections, and sores. You can use sage oil as lotion, for warm aroma bath, or as perfume for best effects.

The Chamomile Oil. This oil is popular for its calming ability which is why this is also known to heal insomnia, infections, depression, pain, fever, gas, convulsions, and skin allergies. For this oil to give good effects, you can use it as a diffuser for insomnia sufferers or apply on hot or cold compress for pain sufferers, particularly those who suffer stomach ache.

The Eucalyptus Oil. This essential oil can help heal respiratory problems, pain like muscle pain, wounds, cavities and other dental problems, stress, skin diseases, intestinal germs and even fever. To help achieve the great effects of eucalyptus oil, use it as a diffuser, lotion, blend with other essential oils, or use it as a perfume.

The Cinnamon Oil. This oil heals blood impurities, diabetes, infections, bad breath, bleeding, pain, indigestion, menstrual discomfort and respiratory problems. It is best used as a diffuser either by dripping the oil into water or through the use of a cinnamon scented candle.

The Ginger Oil. This oil is not only used for cooking but it is also known to heal stomach problems whether they are stomach aches, etc. It also heals symptoms of food poisoning, nausea and vomiting, heart ailments, stress, kidney problems, impotency, respiratory problems, and hair care problems. Ginger oil is best used as a diffuser, oil for massage, and steam inhalation.

The Hyssop Oil. As one of the oldest essential oils, this oil has the ability to heal dental and digestive problems, rheumatism, infections, respiratory problems, wounds, urinary problems and gases. Hyssop oil is best used as massage oil, diffuser, oil for aromatherapy bath, or simply apply on the affected area for faster healing.

The Jasmine Oil. Jasmine oil heals depression, cramps, infections, congestions, asthma, scars, impotence, dysmenorrhea, stress, cough, tumors, etc. The oil of the jasmine flower is best used in bath water, as steam inhalation for coughs, diffuser for fertility problems and calming nervousness, and massage oil for injuries and muscle pains.

The Lavender Oil. Lavender oil is an oil used to heal headaches, insomnia, anxiety, urinary disorders, sprains and pains, respiratory disorders, treat hypertension, digestive problems, hair lice infestations, wounds, cuts and burns, and insect bites. This oil is popularly used as an ointment for burns, stings, and itching; as lotions for healing chapped skin, and diffuser for allergies and respiratory problems.

The Myrrh Oil. Myrrh oil is used for healing microbial and viral infections, dental problems, cough and respiratory diseases, breathing trouble and congestion, fungal infections, as well as wounds and cuts. Myrrh oil is best used by direct application and as massage oil.

The Oregano Oil. Oregano oil is used to heal viral infections like mumps, small pox, etc. It can also heal bacterial and fungal infections like urinary tract infections, skin diseases, etc. It can also treat signs of aging like wrinkles, etc. as well as heal parasite infections. It can also heal allergies and digestive problems. To achieve the benefits of oregano oil, this is best used as topical creams and lotions as well as internal or oral use.

The Lemon Oil. Lemon oil can heal stress, insomnia, stomach ailments, dizziness, obesity, fever, pimples and other skin disorders, asthma, cough and other respiratory ailments. The effects of lemon oil can be achieved through steam inhalation, tonic or juice, or for use directly on affected area.

The Patchouli Oil. This essential oil is good for healing depression, wounds, impotency and fertility problems, inflammations, dental problems, fever, allergies, cough, scars, and parasite infections. This essential oil is best used as massage oil, lotion, and shampoo.

The Rosemary Oil. Rosemary oil heals indigestion, bad breath, depression, dandruff, memory loss, skin dryness, pain and respiratory problems. Rosemary Oil can be used for aromatherapy bath, steam inhalation, and shampoo.

The Lemongrass Oil. This essential oil heals muscle and joint pain, food poisoning, high fever, wounds, body odor, depression, urinary disorders, nervous disorders, insomnia, fungal infections, and digestive problems. You can use lemongrass oil through direct application on affected area especially in fungal infections, lotions, steam inhalation, massage oils and as insect repellant.

The Sandalwood Oil. This essential oil is essential for healing wounds and cuts, viral infections, cramps and aches, fever, muscle, gum, and skin contractions, scars, urinary tract infections, gases, cough and colds, digestive problems, circulatory and respiratory problems as well as anxiety and depression,. For best results, use sandalwood oil as warm sandalwood bath, vaporizer, lotions and creams.

The Peppermint Oil. Peppermint oil has healing properties for the treatment of indigestion, dental problems, respiratory problems, nausea, irritable bowel, headache, urinary tract infections, pain, as well as dandruff. Its effects can be achieved when this oil is used as massage oil, steam inhalation, tonic, and aromatherapy bath or as a diffuser.

The Tea Tree Oil. Tea tree oil is popularly known as treatment for bacterial infections either in urinary tract, stomach, intestines, etc., wounds and cuts, microbial infections like malaria and boils, viral infections like colds, mumps, as well as cough, parasite infections and fungal infections. To achieve its aroma and healing benefits, use tea tree oil through direct application on affected area with the use of cotton, use it as gargle solution, dandruff shampoo, steam inhalation, and through aromatherapy bath.

The Vanilla Oil. Vanilla oil can heal memory loss, erectile dysfunction, cancers, wrinkles, fever, impotency, depression, hypertension, stress, as well as insomnia.

Vanilla oil can be used as a beauty mask, aromatherapy bath, and as a massage oil to reap its benefits.

The Pine Oil. Pine needle extracts can be used for healing skin and facial diseases like pimples, eczema, etc., pain due to arthritis and rheumatism, stress and infections, wounds and injuries as well as respiratory problems. Pine oil is best used as tonic or tea, shampoo, vaporizer, and lotion.

The Wintergreen Oil. This essential oil is a great solution for healing all types of pains, cramps, diarrhea, stress, cough, digestive problems, bad breath and dental problems, nausea and fatigue and kidney infections. For best effects, use wintergreen oil as massage oils and creams as well as mouthwash.

The Thyme Oil. Thyme oil heals cramps and aches, infections, sores, urinary disorders, cough, wounds, vomiting, injuries, nausea, hypertension, intestinal worms, congestion, bad breath and body odor. Thyme oil is best used for aromatherapy bath for relaxation or by spraying it all over the house. You can even enjoy its effects by creating a thyme oil diffuser.

The Nutmeg Oil. This essential oil can heal pain, cramps (either menstrual cramps or leg cramps), hypertension, asthma, indigestion, stress, bad breath, aching gums, heart problems, kidney infections, and liver infections. Nutmeg oil benefits can best be achieved when you use this essential oil as massage oil, as a diffuser, or even apply it on your nice, warm aromatherapy bath.

The Marjoram Oil. Marjoram oil heals headache, spasms, impotency, toothache, cold, cramps, measles, flatulence, arthritis, bacterial infections, rheumatism, hypertension, as well as fungal infections. Marjoram's benefits are best achieved by using this oil as a diffuser for your home, massage oil for pains, as well as steam inhalation for asthma and respiratory problems.

Now, just because essential oils are good for you and has many essential benefits, it does not mean that you can just use them without awareness of the different essential oil precautions. Essential oils differ and skin types differ as well. What could be good and best for one may not be good and best for another. Failing to bear in mind some precautions may put you in grave danger instead of being healed by these essential oils. Knowing and abiding by these precautions can help you know what and what not to do with regards to essential oils.

Chapter 3. Essential Oil Recipes

Recipe for Insomnia and Good Sleep

Aromatherapy therapy can help people that have difficulty in sleeping. There are aromatherapies recipes that could help calm a restless body and mind plus induce sleep. You need 2 drops of rosewood oil, 2 drops of bergamot and 2 drops of ylang ylang. Combine these ingredients to make a strong and fragrant mixture. Rosewood and ylang ylang have a distinct fragrance that will help soothe ails and pains. The smell will also help calm a restless person down plus will also induce sleep in people having difficulty in sleeping. This aromatherapy fragrance will also be a perfect scent on your pillow, bed sheets or on your curtain. Place this oil blends on your curtains, bedding or blankets so your room will smell great and relaxing.

Daytime Aromatherapy Oil Blend

Aromatherapy will also help calm during the day. This is a blend that will uplift your spirit and get you going especially when you are tired and sleepy. You need about 2 drops of geranium oil, 2 drops of rosewood and another 2 drops of bergamot. Combine these three ingredients and you will get a fragrant oil that you may wear as a perfume. Warm the oils up with the use of a water bath and you get a gentle massage oil. You may use this oil in a relaxing massage. Place a few drops on your temples, at the nape of your neck or over the scalp. This oil may also be used as a body massage on the back, the legs, calves and on the hands and feet.

Aromatherapy for Insomnia

Insomnia may be a result of stress, anxiety and pain. Insomnia could lead to depression and even a variety of physiologic condition. Aromatherapy will help curb insomnia and this essential oil blend is made of 3 drops of lavender oil and a drop of sage oil. Use a plain, unscented cream as a base and mix the drops of oils completely. You may place this cream over the body or you may also place the drops of oils into a warm bath. Soak for at least 20 minutes. You should take a warm bath soak just before you go to sleep. Take a warm bath each night just before you retire, you will soon feel relaxed and more eager to go to sleep. This aromatherapy oil blend may also be used to reduce sleeping disorders like interrupted sleep or sleep irregularity.

Aromatherapy Massage Recipe

Aromatherapy oils may be blended together to create an aromatherapy massage base. Massage has been used since ancient times also through the use of essential oils. This recipe calls for 4 drops of lavender oil, a drop of petitgrain and a drop of Frankincense. Blend the three aromatic oils together and you will be able to create a massage base. Massage all over the body or place a few drops of the massage base in a warm bath soak. Massage this over the temples, the scalp and the neck. You may also use this oil blend for a shoulder massage, arm massage or for a back massage after a long and tiring day. If you are going to use this oil in a warm bath soak make sure that you maintain the temperature of your bath water. Stay on the tub as long as you can and then rinse off. Your skin will feel and smell great the entire night long which is perfect for people that have sleep difficulties.

Calming Aromatherapy Oil

You may want to try lavender oil as a massage oil. Lavender is a natural oil that has amazing calming properties that will keep your nerves still and will help you promote sleep. Lavender tea is known to relax a person and then make him feel ready to go to sleep. Use quality lavender oil from a reputable supplier about 4 drops of the oil. There are several ways to use lavender oil; you may place 4 drops in a tablespoon of milk or cream. Place the mixture in a warm bath and then stir. Soak for as long as you want to calm you down. You may also add the oil to a massage cream or oil base and then place the oil over a diffuser and then place in a place near your bed in your bedroom. The heat from the diffuser will slowly evaporate the oil and will make you feel calm and sleepy in no time at all. Lavender is also available in tea form. Pick pure lavender tea from a reputable supplier. Steep your warm tea for about 15 minutes all the while taking deep breaths of the heavenly lavender fumes. Drink this tea just before you go to sleep or you may take it when you feel anxious or stressed even in the middle of the day. However you should never take lavender tea if you plan to drive or to operate machinery since you will feel light and sleepy afterwards.

Aromatherapy Recipe for Muscle Pain

Almost everyone has experienced having muscle pain especially after long hours of physical activity. What happens is the muscles of the body part used for the activity becomes strained and may even become torn after frequent use. Aromatherapy is effective in the relief of pain. Oils such as lavender oil and rosemary are two of the most common oils to use.

Mix about 2 drops of lavender oil and 2 drops of rosemary. Place the blended oils to a carrier oil and then massage over the affected area. For instance, if you are suffering from leg pain you may use this muscle pain oil recipe. Warm your hands first by clapping or rubbing them together. Place a few drops of oil on your palms and then slowly massage the oil over your legs. Use long strokes on your legs; work on the oil slowly and carefully to increase blood circulation over the area. Place an elastic bandage over the area if you wish.

Pain may also be a result of injury such as a sprain, torn ligament or a fracture so before using aromatherapy oils for a massage assess the area first. If you suspect a fracture, immobilize the area with the use of a splint and a bandage. Take the person to a medical facility for treatment.

Aromatherapy Oils Blend as a Pre-Exercise Massage

Fitness enthusiasts recommend using a pre- exercise or sports massage to prevent injuries. Aromatherapy oil will make the area warm and ready to be subjected to strenuous physical stress. The most common combination of oils to make a pre-sports massage are rosemary, lavender and eucalyptus. Simply place 2 drops of each on your palm and apply to your entire body with special attention to your legs, upper extremities. Do you plan to exercise a specific part of your body so you can spot tone? This blend of aromatherapy oils will help reduce pains and strain after you exercise. You should perform exercise that will prepare your body for the strenuous physical activity ahead like jogging, jumping jacks, brisk walking and stretching exercises.

Aromatherapy Therapy Oil Blends for Post-Exercise

It's important to reduce pain and to assess any muscle injuries after a very strenuous exercise regimen. You can do this by applying a selection of aromatherapy oils that will help reduce pain, swelling and soreness. The best selection of oils is rosemary, lavender and eucalyptus. Use 2 drops of rosemary that will help reduce inflammation and pain, 2 drops of lavender to induce calmness and 2 drops of eucalyptus that will help deliver warmth on any affected area. Warm your hands first and then place the oils on your palms and apply these on your skin. Use long and kneading strokes over the legs and arms while using firm and pressing strokes on large parts of the body like the shoulders.

As you use these oil blends for post-exercise, you will be able to assess for any injuries. If there is acute pain, do not continue your massage but instead immobilize the area with a bandage and splint. Call for help immediately.

Aromatherapy Oils for Poor Concentration and Anxiety

Sometimes there are situations that could make us feel anxious, stressed and reduce our concentration. Aromatherapy could help reduce these negative symptoms and return our calm and peaceful state of mind. There are a few oils that can do this and one of them is lavender. Lavender is available in essence form, in packets of tea and in lavender perfume. If you feel anxious, prepare a warm cup of lavender tea. Allow the tea bag to steep for about 15 minutes all the while smelling the lavender essence.

If you have a diffuser, place about two drops of lavender and let the scent fill the room. You may also spray lavender perfume on your bed, curtains and on your blanket so you will feel calmer and ready to sleep at the end of the day.

Chapter 4. Essential Oil Precautions

Patch test is necessary for allergic reactions. Not all skin types may be comfortable with certain essential oils and this could cause allergic reactions and irritations instead of healing. To avoid this, it is important to conduct a patch test first or applying a bit of essential oil on the skin just to test whether your skin will react negatively to it or not.

Too much is a hazard. Using essential oils topically, orally or through inhalation should be done moderately. You don't need to put too much especially if you are not yet sure of how your skin or your body will react.

Store essential oils out of children's reach. Children mostly have no idea how to use essential oils and they could be in danger if they use these oils improperly. So, it is a must for these oils to be out of children's reach or if they need these oils' benefits, they must be assisted by their parents.

Store essential oils away from fire and heat. Essential oils may not be like other oils but they are also highly flammable. With this, when exposed to heat or fire they could explode and cause fire accidents.

Consult the doctor or experts when it comes to essential oils. The most important precaution to bear in mind is to always consult the experts when it comes to using essential oils. You could be in a condition where you are not sure whether some oils are advised. You could be pregnant, diabetic, etc. and certain oils may not be advised to be used in your condition. This way you need experts to advise you whether certain oils are good for you or not. Also, you need to consult experts regarding the administration or application of essential oils. There are essential oils that can be administered orally, while there some that are for external use only and there are also some people who want to use it for aromatherapy. Consulting experts first will let you know how to use certain essential oils.

Conclusion

To sum up, essential oils indeed have essential uses and benefits which is why they are called essential oils. From physical benefits, emotional benefits, to mental benefits and stress-busting benefits, essential oils are getting popular in the market nowadays because of these. They are considered nature's best gift because they are natural products and unlike synthetic products out there, they are much safer to be used because they do not contain chemicals. While they offer great effects, they offer lesser to no side effects provided you choose the right products.

However, since your safety can be at risk with the improper and careless use and administration of these essential oils, it is essential to follow essential oil precautions. As long as you follow the necessary precautions when using essential oils, nothing can hinder you from reaping the benefits of these oils.

Thank You Page

I want to personally thank you for reading my book. I hope you found information in this book useful and I would be very grateful if you could leave your honest review about this book. I certainly want to thank you in advance for doing this.

www.ingramcontent.com/pod-product-compliance
Lightning Source LLC
Chambersburg PA
CBHW060349290526
45791CB00004B/1599